40 Days of Faith and Fitness: A Devotional Journal

Marsha Apsley

A heartfelt thank you to Dr. Beth Brombosz. Without her assistance I would've never realized this dream of putting these devotions into the book you now hold in your hands. She walked me through every step of this process and gave me the confidence to take this leap of faith.

Thank you also goes to Nicole Culver and Blogger to Business group. Nicole has created a supportive community of female entrepreneurs who cheer each other on through the highs and lows of growing a business. These girls let me cry on their shoulders and have been my biggest fans.

CONTENTS

Marsha Apsley

ACKNOWLEDGMENTS

Special thank you to these women for reviewing my book and giving me valuable feedback.

Dr. Beth Brombosz
www.bloggertoauthor.com

Tammy Etter

Kat Downs
www.crunchykat.com

Lindsey Janeiro
www.nutritiontofit.com

INTRODUCTION

As far back as I can remember, I've always loved devotions. I'd get a new one every year. I always had one by my bed or with my Bible.

I gave my heart to Jesus when I was 9, and I've had regular daily quiet times since then. At about the same age, I started struggling with insecurities and body image. It essentially became a lifelong battle until about the time I was turning 40. Some of that journey is shared in the following pages.

So why tell you those things? That's how this devotional came to be. I prayed often about my insecurities and weight loss issues, and I searched for scriptures and all kinds of encouragement, but I always returned to diets, weight loss pills, and quick fixes. Eventually I totally gave this all to God, and I found freedom. I started writing the verses down and what they meant to me.

The season of Lent is a special time because a few years ago I joined an online community called 40 Days of Prayer and Fitness. This was another step in that freedom process. The next year I hosted my own 40 days group because I wanted to give back for what I had received the year before. And then the following year I was thinking about what to do for Lent, and I was prompted to go to my documents and count how many verses I had logged. Sure enough there were nearly 40 at the time. That's when

I finished them up, put them in an email series, and invited some women to go along with me on a 40 Days of Faith and Fitness journey.

The devotions were well-received. Each day meant a new verse, some devotional content, a prayer, and an action step.

Now, you have those devotions in your hands along with a journal page to document how that verse speaks to your life and how you take that action step and the results of it.

For too long, I cried tears over the reflection in the mirror instead of seeing the woman God created me to be. For too long, I was bound up with negative thoughts about myself and a focus on losing weight in order to be happy and feel good.

It is my prayer that no girl or woman struggle for as long as I did. I now know that my healthy life must be built on a firm foundation of faith.

How is that done? By knowing God's word and what He says about me and my body and then putting it into action. Some days it requires all the faith I have to believe that I am "fearfully and wonderfully made." Other days I get that glimpse that I truly am royalty and a daughter of a King.

May these devotions speak into your life and help you build your fit life on a firm foundation.

HOW TO USE

Each day includes a scripture, devotional content, prayer, and an action step.

Following the action step, you'll find a journal page. This is for you to use however you wish, or perhaps not at all.

Some ways you may consider using your journal page:

- You may want to write down how you took the action for the day.

- Maybe you'd like to write your own prayer.

- You may even want to spend some quiet time and ask God how He wants you to respond to the day's verse and content.

My prayer for you is that at the end of these 40 days you will become more aware of God's love for you just as you are. In addition, I hope that you will find tools to help you live a sustainable healthy life, one that honors the unique body you've been entrusted with.

Enjoy the journey. I'm praying for you Beautiful One.

V

DAY 1

"Do not remember the former things, nor consider the things of old. Behold, I will do a new thing, now it shall spring forth; shall you not know it? I will even make a road in the wilderness and river in the desert." Isaiah 43:18-19 (NKJV)

It's a new day! It's not time to look back at what you've tried and failed at. Today is the time to start and move forward from here on out!

When you make the decision to start living a healthy life or make improvements in your health and fitness, I know that one of the things that seem to paralyze you is what you've already tried and failed.

I know that it can be easy to look back at what worked and what didn't work and wonder why it worked then but why it can't work now. Or wonder if although it didn't work then it may work now.

Do you know how much time I've wasted scouring food diaries and journals that I would keep? I'd log calories and exercise and get on a weight loss streak and then I'd gain. And I didn't know why. I didn't think that I had changed anything when it came to my eating or exercise. But even still, I'd spend an hour going through my food logs trying to figure out where I had gone wrong and what I needed to do to change it.

No more!!! We weren't made to look back. We aren't supposed to get stuck in the old places.

This is a new day! God's ready to do a new thing. Are you ready?

Your approach is going to be different because you're going to go at this keeping your eyes on Him. You're going to commit this process to Him and honor the unique way that He made **you**.

Prayer: Dear God, I'm ready for a new day! I'm not looking back. Please help me only to look forward toward You and the path that You are making for me. In Jesus' Name, Amen.

Action Step: Commit today to only look forward. No looking back. Let go of the things that once dragged you down. Write this verse on a notecard or in a journal with the date beside it. Sign it as your commitment to being ready for a new thing!

Journal

DAY 2

"Do you not know that your body is the temple of the Holy Spirit, who is in you, whom you have received from God, you are not your own? For you were bought at a price; therefore glorify God in your body and in your spirit which are God's." 1 Corinthians 6:19-20 (NKJV)

You are priceless. You were created with care and purpose. You are an original.

Do you care for your body as if you are a temple? As if you are priceless and have been created with care and purpose?

If you are a Christ-follower, the Holy Spirit dwells in you. Is He comfortable in your skin? Do you care for yourself, your spirit and your body, in a way that honors the Lord?

These are questions to consider as you move through the coming days. It's time to see yourself as Christ sees you and to begin to honor Him by honoring the body He has given you.

Prayer: Lord, thank You for the care and concern with which You created me. Help me to honor You with my body. I want Your Holy Spirit to feel comfortable in me. Amen.

Action: Walk tall today. You are royalty. When you make choices with what you are eating and drinking and the media you are consuming, consider yourself as a temple

4

and only consume those things which will honor that.

Journal

DAY 3

"These things I have spoken to you, that in Me you may have peace. In the world you will have tribulation; but be of good cheer, I have overcome the world." John 16:33 (NKJV)

Peace.

One of the definitions on Dictionary.com is this: freedom of the mind from annoyance, distraction, anxiety, an obsession, etc. When it comes to our health and fitness, I believe that this is the perfect definition. Let's look at it…

Freedom of the mind…isn't that what we're seeking? I know I was. All my years of struggle with my weight and body image was in my mind. It distracted me from everything else. I was anxious about what I would eat or when I would exercise. I was obsessed with how I looked, what I weighed, how many calories were in something. And all I wanted at the end of the day was freedom. I just wanted to be free from these thoughts and worries and obsessions.

I wanted peace.

Sure, I was a Christian. I accepted Jesus into my heart as a young girl, but I didn't let Him have every area. I didn't think this really mattered much to Him. I was selfish to want to be pretty and skinny and to want boys to like me. I didn't realize that He came for me and paid the ultimate sacrifice for me and was interested in *everything* about me. He had the peace that I needed, but I had to accept that peace.

It took a long time for me to experience freedom in this area…a very long time! I was nearly 40 when I finally started seeing that I could be free. I didn't need to live in this constant state of anxiety with obsessive thoughts flitting through my head all the time.

Society seemed to shout "I have the answer over here. Just take this pill." "You need to look like this to get a boyfriend." In the midst of that noise is Christ and the peace that only He can offer. Yes, we'll have these messages bombarding us until the end of time, but we don't have to buy into them. We don't have to let them distract us from the peace that is ours if only we'll accept it.

Prayer: Dear God, I want to be free. I want to be free from the anxiety and the obsessive thoughts that are taking over my mind. I know that You have already bought my peace and You give it freely. Here I am Lord; please bless me with Your peace. In the midst of the noise and the hard days, please shower me with Your peace. I'm asking this in Your name, Amen.

Action Step: Turn off all the noise. Step away from your electronic devices and get quiet in His presence. Experience His peace firsthand.

Journal

DAY 4

"All things are lawful for me, but all things are not helpful. All things are lawful for me, but I will not be brought under the power of any." 1 Corinthians 6:12 (NKJV)

There is another version of this same concept in 1 Corinthians 10:23: *"Everything is permissible but not everything is beneficial."*

I love the freedom found in this verse. But in this same verse we find boundaries. Everything is permissible. We can have or do anything, BUT not everything is beneficial. And that is where the work comes in and the boundaries get set up.

Boundaries provide safety. We let our children run and play outside, but not in the street. We let them go into the backyard where they are safe within the fence.

We are free to drive on the open roads, but there are speed limits and lanes that we have to stay inside to keep us safe.

When we are embarking on a healthy lifestyle, we need to figure out how our bodies respond to certain foods and exercise. All food is permissible. But I'm finding that my body doesn't respond well to dairy products. Dairy is perfectly good, but for me it's not beneficial. My stomach hurts when I eat it.

With the popularity of gluten-free diets, we know that some people truly do not respond well to too much gluten in their diet. Again, it is permissible and perfectly okay for many people, but if gluten leaves you feeling bloated and your stomach in knots, then it's not beneficial for you.

This process may take a little while; however, once you begin to pay attention to YOU, you'll know what you need to do to honor your unique body.

Prayer: Lord, show me what is beneficial for my body. I know that I have access to many things, but I want to operate within the safety of the boundaries You have set for me. Amen.

Action: Become a detective of YOU. Don't follow someone else's restrictive diet because you think it should work for you. Figure out what is beneficial for you. And then honor that. Stay within those boundaries. Start journaling or taking notes about what you're eating and how you're feeling afterwards. Monitor energy levels, how well you sleep, how your body feels. Take positive action based on what you find.

Journal

DAY 5

"Commit to the Lord whatever you do and He will establish your plan." Proverbs 16:3 (NIV)

I'm a Type A personality. I like lists and goals and agendas. I have the family calendar pretty much memorized. I live by a schedule and always have a plan.

When it comes to health and fitness, I've followed all kinds of diets and programs. I've read magazine after magazine and have clipped articles on everything from what to eat and when and how to exercise to every sort of recipe imaginable.

For the longest time, I separated my faith and my fitness. Yes, I prayed the Lord would help me lose weight and like myself (in that order…weight had to come off first, right??). But then I pored through books and magazines for diets, supplements, exercises, etc., that claimed to help me achieve the body I was hoping for.

It wasn't until just a few years ago that I realized that I had to commit this fitness plan to the Lord. I had to seek His input on what was best for my body. It wasn't something I could come up with on my own and then hope He'd bless. HE wanted to be the one to show me.

I had to commit to the Lord the changes I needed in my body and mind. Then He would help me with that plan.

It took nearly 40 years, but I got there.

Oh there are many times I try to go by my plan, but I quickly realize that I have to let Him be my planner!

Prayer: Lord, I want to change my thoughts towards my body. I want to live a healthy and fit life. I need You to show me the plan that is right for me. Lead me on this journey. I trust that with You I can do this. Amen.

Action Step: If you have a plan written out or a book you're reading or trying to follow, literally lay it out before the Lord. Pray over it. Ask Him if this is where He's really leading you. If it is, then stick to it. If not, then ask Him to show you a better way.

Journal

DAY 6

"This is the day the Lord has made; we will rejoice and be glad in it." Psalm 118:24 (NKJV)

Every day when I wake up, I say the verse above. I thank the Lord for another day He's given me. It's a great way to get my focus on *whose* day this is.

Oh, there are good days and bad days. And my attitude has much to do with it. But if I don't approach each day with this intention, I don't even have a chance of making it what He wants it to be.

These days aren't our days. He has given them to us. He has allowed you and me yet another day to be here. And what am I doing with this day? Am I rejoicing? Am I looking to Him to lead me? Am I intentionally doing what He's called me to do? Or, am I complaining? Am I noting everything that is wrong about the day?

How are you going to approach today? I hope you say, "Rejoice!"

Prayer: Lord, this is the day You have made. I *will* rejoice and be glad in it. Thank You for giving me the breath in my lungs. I will use it to praise You. Amen.

Action Step: Put on some uplifting music and have a dance party before the Lord.

Journal

DAY 7

"For as he thinks in his heart, so is he." Proverbs 23:7 (NKJV)

There are so many concepts before and after this verse in chapter 23, and they all seem to sum up my life's story.

There is caution against gluttony and an unhealthy focus on food. And then there is a call out to parents to instruct and to children to listen to their parents. My testimony starts as a Jesus-loving young girl consumed with how she looked. I watched my mom struggle with her weight, and she desperately did not want me to deal with the same issues. Unfortunately that made me (and her) hyper-focused on it, and I began to believe I was fat, ugly, not good enough, and that I would never find anyone to love me.

For as (s)he thinks in his(her) heart, so is (s)he.

I struggled with what the doctors would call a "nervous stomach." I was painfully shy and introverted and worried about everything. I worried about what people thought of me, of how I looked to others, if anyone would ever love me enough to marry me.

For as (s)he thinks in his(her) heart, so is (s)he.

By the time I was in 6th grade, I was following Weight Watchers and eating pretzels and drinking milk for my lunch all because I thought I was fat and would never catch the eye of someone who would want to love me.

For as (s)he thinks in his(her) heart, so is (s)he.

Fast-forward to college, more feelings of not being good enough, not thin enough, not fit enough. (Yes, the focus was solely on my looks!) I dabbled with forms of purging (laxatives and over-exercising) to try to lose weight.

For as (s)he thinks in his(her) heart, so is (s)he.

Finally I found a man who showed some interest, and I married him. For nearly 5 years we struggled to make it work, but I still had all the baggage of my worth and my own identity. We weren't able to make the marriage last.

For as (s)he thinks in his(her) heart, so is (s)he.

As I stated in the beginning, I've followed Jesus from my early years. I cried and struggled through all of this. I laid it at His feet and picked it back up more times than I can count. I prayed and prayed that He'd make me beautiful and that I'd see that reflection in the mirror, but I just would never let His message of true love penetrate my heart.

For as (s)he thinks in his(her) heart, so is (s)he.

As my adult life went on, I managed the insecurities. Yes, I'd cry over numbers on the scales and the reflection in the mirror, but I got better at living with it. I rather resigned myself to the fact that this would be my life…restless, unsettled, dissatisfied with my physical body.

For as (s)he thinks in his(her) heart, so is (s)he.

But then I hit a fork in the road just as I was about to turn 40. I read the book <u>Made to Crave</u> by Lysa TerKeurst. In one section she quoted a verse when God told Moses "You have circled this mountain long enough." Hmmm…40 years in the desert. I was nearly 40. God was telling me it was TIME. Let's turn north.

For as (s)he thinks in his(her) heart, so is (s)he.

Oh, it wasn't like flipping a switch and now I knew and believed everything written in His word about how I'm "fearfully and wonderfully made" and "loved with an everlasting love." But it was the catalyst. Slowly, I began to let go of my insecurities. Slowly I began to take the chance at believing that maybe I was okay. Slowly the thoughts in my heart began to change.

For as (s)he thinks in his(her) heart, so is (s)he.

What's in your heart? Are you believing God? Are you taking Him at His word?

From a young age, I knew I was a child of God. I knew it in my head, but it took me many years to get it in my heart and to know that I was perfect just the way I was.

Let His word penetrate your heart today. Take Him at His word.

For as (s)he thinks in his(her) heart, so is (s)he.

I am a fearfully and wonderfully created daughter of the King.

Prayer: Thank You for making me unique, Lord. Help me to know this truth deep down in my heart. I ask this in Your name, Amen.

Action Step: Stand in front of the mirror and say "I am a fearfully and wonderfully created daughter of the King."

Journal

DAY 8

"Not that I have already attained, or am already perfected; but I press on, that I may lay hold of that for which Christ Jesus has also laid hold of me." Philippians 3:12 (NKJV)

I'm not there yet; I'm not perfect, but I press on toward that which Christ has called me.

We're all a work in progress. Until we meet Jesus, we'll never be perfect. We all have issues that we struggle with and we work to improve, but our insecurities always seem to sneak up.

I'm not a fan of transformation pictures that show bare midriffs. But I am a fan of transformations that happen on the inside. You see, you can't really photograph those, but that's what this verse is talking about.

We're pressing into Him and we're changing on the inside. It happens on our health and fitness journey. It's not about showcasing the body change, although that can and will happen. The change that matters is what happens on the inside, the change that happens in our thinking and in the way we view ourselves. We begin to see ourselves as fearfully and wonderfully made. We embrace the unique way He created us and the calling that He's placed on us.

Press into Him. Press forward on the journey that He's leading you.

Prayer: Lord, thank You for sticking with me. Thank You

for the work You're doing in my life. Thank You for not giving up on me. Make me all that You want me to be so that You can be glorified in me. Please change me from the inside out. Amen.

Action Step: Look back at some pictures of yourself. How have you changed? Maybe you've made changes physically, but I want you to look on the inside of that person you're looking at. Only you know the transformations that have happened. Thank Him for where you've come. If there are changes yet to be made, spend time asking Him to help you make those changes.

Journal

DAY 9

"Have mercy on me, O Lord, for I am weak. O Lord heal me for my bones are troubled." Psalm 6:2 (NKJV)

I found this verse when I needed healing in my feet. I was getting ready to run a half marathon and an unexplained injury popped up in my feet. I needed healing to make it through the 13.1 miles.

I know we're not supposed to take scripture out of context and make it what we want it to be. But I sat before the Lord and prayed for a specific scripture that I could hold onto through the run. He led me to this. I wrote it on a notecard and recited it during the race. I ran without pain or complications.

Sister, God's word is living and active. When we open it, He will speak to us. He will use it to speak into our unique lives. I am weak. I need His word. I need Him. He is there. He has a word for me. In fact, I'm sure there are many words that He has for me that I've failed to hear because I've rush through my daily quiet time.

But He is there. Always there. Waiting. Patiently. Ready to speak when I'm ready to listen.

Do you need a word from Him? He has the answers.

Prayer: Lord, help me take the time to prepare my heart and listen. Speak a word into my life today. Thank You for being the same yesterday, today, and forever. Amen.

Action Step: Grab your Bible and sit before the Lord. Tell Him what's in your heart. Ask Him to give you a personal word. And listen. He will show you.

Journal

DAY 10

"Do you not know that you are the temple of God, and that the Spirit of God dwells in you? If anyone defiles the temple of God, God will destroy him. For the temple of God is holy, which temple you are." I Corinthians 3:16-17 (NKJV)

YOU are a temple. You have been carefully crafted and created.

I would love to go overseas and visit places like France and Italy and see all the amazing buildings and structures. Even now, I can just picture walking in very slowly and carefully and then gazing around.

If I were able to go there, do you think I'd slop in with muddy shoes or run down the aisle screaming or leave my trash behind? Of course not. I'd go in with awe and reverence. I'd be quiet and probably step lightly. I certainly would be careful not to drop any trash. In fact, I wouldn't even take anything in with me that could contaminate the place in any way.

YOU are a temple. What do you put in it? What do you allow in it? What kind of food? What kind of words do you speak to yourself?

I first heard this from Michelle Myers. She remarked "Are you going to treat your body like a temple or a trash can?" That's something to think about.

Are you going to fill your body with good food and uplifting words? Or are you going to eat the scraps off the children's plates so the food doesn't go into the trash can? Are you going to speak to yourself with kind words or are you going to look in the mirror and point at all the flaws?

When you visit a temple or a beautiful building, do you stand there and tell your husband about the cobweb way up in the corner or the chipped paint on the baseboard? I doubt you even see those things. (If they're even there!) You just see the majesty of the place and appreciate all the work that has gone into it.

So it should be with you. You are a temple, not a trash can. Start treating yourself as such.

Prayer: Lord, thank You for taking time to create me perfectly the way You did. I want my body to be a welcome place for You to live. Help me to treat it with love and respect and not dismiss it as a trash can. Amen.

Action Step: When you find yourself eating or drinking something, or saying something to yourself, stop and ask "Am I treating myself like a temple or a trash can?" One clear way for me is at meal clean up. Have you found yourself eating a leftover instead of throwing it in the trash just so "it doesn't go to waste"? Do you see how that makes you the trash can? Just throw it away.

Journal

DAY 11

"No discipline seems pleasant at the time, but painful. Later on, however, it produces a harvest of righteousness and peace for those who have been trained by it. Therefore, strengthen your feeble arms and weak knees, and make straight paths for your feet, so that the lame may not be disabled, but rather healed." Hebrews 12:11-13 (NIV)

I know you get tired of living a healthy lifestyle sometimes. It's not always easy to make the right food choice or drink all the water or move every day. But those are the days that the discipline and the training pays off.

If you are just starting out, that means you're going to have to dig deep to commit to the training. At first it will require self-discipline and commitment. But it'll pay off.

Maybe you've been living the healthy lifestyle for years, but you're feeling tired, maybe even getting bored. Remember how good it feels to know you're doing the right thing, how good it feels to make the healthy choices.

This journey isn't always easy. Life, in general, can be hard. But we know that there is more to the here and now. We know that we have a Savior that has made a path for us. He is our healer. He is our strength when we are weary.

If you are feeling tired or feel as if you just can't make another healthy choice, I urge you to keep at it. Stick with it! It's worth it.

Having the energy to play with your children and grandchildren is worth it.

Being able to take a walk and move freely without getting out of breath is worth it.

Feeling clean and healthy is worth it.

Honoring your body because you are a temple is worth it.

Prayer: Lord help me, especially on days like today when I'm tired and struggling. I know that You will bless my obedience. I know that I will be better for making the hard but healthy choices. Please give me strength today. I ask this in Your name, Amen.

Action Step: Go for a walk. Play with your little ones or grandchildren. Celebrate any progress that you've already made and commit to moving forward.

- Journal

DAY 12

"Trust in the Lord, and do good; dwell in the land, and feed on His faithfulness. Delight yourself also in the Lord, and He shall give you the desires of your heart. Commit your way to the Lord, trust also in Him, and He shall bring it to pass." Psalm 37:3-5 (NIV)

Several years ago I heard this passage preached, specifically "Delight yourself in the Lord, and He will give you the desires of your heart." I can't remember the speaker, but he explained it like this: If you are following the Lord and seeking Him, *He* will put desires in your heart that He wants you to pursue.

This is not a verse saying that if you want a new car, God will give it to you. Or if we are ready to get married, God will drop a man in front of us.

It means that if we are laser-focused on following Christ, you can be sure that when a strong desire is in our heart, He's put it there.

If you're wondering what your calling is, He'll put a passion in your heart. If you're at a crossroads, He will speak into your heart which way to go.

So when you hear "follow your heart" or "trust your heart," you can do this *if* you're seeking Christ.

And once you take that step in the direction you feel He's leading, commit it to Him and trust that He will be faithful.

Prayer: Lord, I want to follow You. I want what You want for me. My heart is Yours. I open it now. Please fill me with the desires You want for me. Amen.

Action Step: Write out your goals. Then measure them with what is in your heart. Are you seeking Him? Has He put the answer in front of you?

Journal

DAY 13

"Therefore, if anyone is in Christ, he is a new creation; old things have passed away; behold, all things have become new." 2 Corinthians 5:17 (NKJV)

I don't know about you, but I've made so many mistakes. I've screwed up as a wife and as a mom. I've not handled things well as a sister, daughter, or friend. And how many times have I given into eating too much or wallowing in self-pity over something!!

But He can make all things new. He can take anything that I screw up and fix it. If only I give it to Him. But I must give it to Him. I must recognize and repent and TURN. I must address the issue, and then do an about face. I must change direction.

Too often, especially when it comes to messing up with our health and fitness, we tend to wait until Monday to start new and fresh. But what if we messed up on Tuesday?

Trail mix or cookie dough can get me every time!

Well, what if I lose my mind and eat all the cookie dough on Tuesday morning?? Should I wait nearly a week until I start new? I could do much more damage in a week! I could eat A LOT of cookie dough! (and probably get food poisoning!) No, I need to make that change right then and there. Get back on track, back to honoring my body.

Have you ever lost your temper with your child and then felt badly afterwards? I have. So do I just let that go, or do I pray and ask for another chance?

If you are in Christ, He can make it new. He's a loving and forgiving God just waiting for you to reach out to Him for help. In that very instant He will forgive and will help you make all things new...begin mending the relationship or help strengthen that self-discipline.

Do you need a fresh start in some area? Ask Him today.

Prayer: Lord, thank You for fresh starts. Thank You for welcoming me any time and making me new. I lay this struggle at Your feet and I pray for You to make it new. Amen.

Action Step: Take inventory. Is there a change that you need to make? Have you been putting something off? Make today that new day.

Journal

DAY 14

"You have circles this mountain long enough; turn northward."
Deuteronomy 2:3 (AMP)

This verse was THE turning point for me. I was reading <u>Made to Crave</u> by Lysa TerKeurst nearly 5 years ago. I was just about to turn 40. I had been on the journey of finding freedom from the noise in my head, but I was still looking for something, anything to be the magic plan for losing weight and feeling good in my skin.

I was soaking in everything Lysa wrote. So many underlines and stars in this book! Then I came to a section of the book where she began writing about Moses and the Israelites. How God taught them to depend on Him and how it took **40 years!** At that moment, it clicked. I had been wandering for nearly 40 years. And really, friend, that's not much of a stretch. I had spent more of my life on this earth worrying and crying about my weight than I had not. As early as elementary school I was eating dry lettuce and cans of tuna.

As I read this, I made note in the margin of the book - "Soon to be 40. Don't want to wander any longer." Talk about timing! God knew what He was doing. He knew I would read that book on that day and that it would **finally** click.

Marsha, you've been circling this mountain of body image, weight loss, insecurity, comparison, competition, long enough; it's time to turn north.

As I finished that book, I resolved that I was turning North. And I did. I'm still on that journey. I'm not going to try to tell you that I never struggled again. I'm not even going to tell you that I never bought a pill or followed a restrictive diet plan after that. But what I will tell you is that something changed. I was looking in a different direction. I began traveling in a different direction.

It's brought me here. Here to share my story. To this place in my life where I'm living fit AND free. I'm learning how to live a fit and healthy lifestyle that is lived out in freedom and not bondage to numbers or diet plans and programs.

What mountain have you been circling? Are you stuck wandering? Do you feel as if you've been fighting a battle for too long?

Have you been addressing the same struggles and issues and you just can't catch a break? You just can't get past it?

He's telling you, "My Child, it's time to turn North."

Prayer: Dear Lord, I'm ready. I've been wandering far too long. I'm ready to change direction and do it Your way. Here I am. Show me the new direction to go. In Your name I pray, Amen.

Action Step: Draw compass arrows. Plot God on the North arrow. Where are you? What do you need to do to begin moving in the direction He wants you to go?

Journal

DAY 15

"A man's heart plans his way, but the Lord directs his steps."
Proverbs 16:9 (NKJV)

How many times have we tried to do it on our own? Too many for me to count.

How many times have you tried a diet pill that promised quick and lasting results? How many times have you paid for some contraption or program that told you just do this for 10 days and you'll lose 10 pounds?

Years ago I bought "Hot Pants." The claim was that if you wore these to bed, your waist would get smaller while you slept.

Yep, I believed it. I wanted nothing more than to have a flat stomach (I've realized that won't happen in this lifetime!). My Hot Pants are still a joke around the house!

Have you ever thought that the One who made you might have an idea of what would work for you? Have you considered letting *Him* lead and guide you in your health and fitness?

Your faith and your fitness are not things that need to be separate. He wants to be your guide in ALL areas of your life.

No area should be off limits, nor is any area none of His

concern. He is concerned about everything and all of you.

Where do you need His leadership? Surrender to Him completely.

Prayer: Lord please direct my steps. I have hopes, dreams, and desires in my heart, but I want only what You have for me. I'm pausing to let You step in front of me and lead. I trust You, today and every day forward. In Jesus' name, Amen.

Action Step: Write down your dreams and your goals. They can be big or small. It doesn't matter. Then ask yourself if you are allowing Him to take the lead. Surrender and let Him be your guide.

Journal

DAY 16

"Therefore if the Son makes you free, you shall be free indeed."
John 8:36 (NKJV)

Freedom.

It was something I sought for a long time. Before I started picking a word for the year, I had a year in my life that could have easily been defined by this word. It wasn't that I was living in freedom at the time, but I was seeking it daily. If I'd see the word freedom in a book title, I'd pounce on it. If I saw it in the paper or in an article, I'd read it.

I became super focused on this word because I needed it. I didn't exactly know how, but I knew that my focus on my weight and my body was not right. I wanted freedom from the numbers on the scale and the voices that told me I wasn't pretty enough. I wanted to be free from feeling as if I had to count every calorie and calculate every workout and make sure calories in didn't go over calories out.

I wanted to feel good about myself when I walked out the door. But even more, I didn't want to be concerned so much about my appearance. And not in a way that I'd just walk out the door looking terrible. I didn't want to always be wondering what someone else thought of me. I hated being bombarded with thoughts like "I bet she thinks I've gained weight." I didn't want to be comparing myself constantly to all the other women in the room and trying to decide whether I was as thin as or as pretty as someone else.

I just wanted to live. I wanted to be me and be okay with that. I wanted that to be enough. And the thing is, it was enough…it was more than enough…to Christ. He created me. He always thought I was perfect. But I had to believe that. I had to embrace the fact that He came *to set me free.*

I've known Jesus pretty much my entire life. But there was so much He did for me, so much that He had to offer me that I never accepted. He didn't mean for me to live in bondage to these sins of selfishness and pride. Because, let's face it, that's what it was. I was thinking about my weight all the time. I allowed lies to come into my head and tell me things that just weren't true, and I bought them all!!

But He came to set us free. Finally I found that freedom. It was always there for me, but I had to want it. I had to let Him take those chains and release me.

Is there an area of your life that you need to find freedom in? The price has been paid. Let Him unlock the door. Walk out in freedom.

Prayer: Thank You God for the freedom that is found only in You. I don't want to be held hostage any longer by this pain and this hurt. Please set me free. I want to walk freely in the life that You have designed for me. In Jesus' name, Amen.

Action Step: The next time you use your key to unlock your back door or your car door and open it up, think about what area of your life you need to let Him unlock to set you free.

Journal

DAY 17

"Because of the Lord's great love we are not consumed, for his compassions never fail. They are new every morning; great is your faithfulness. I say to myself, 'The Lord is my portion; therefore I will wait for Him.'" Lamentations 3:22-24 (NIV)

New every morning…

Every day is a new day.

Things happen. We mess up. But He is faithful. He gives us a new day. A fresh start.

Does this mean we can just keep messing up and starting over?

Well, He welcomes us with open arms each and every day. But I would suggest that you don't start your day just planning to struggle and eventually concede the day and need to start fresh the next.

Yes, each day is new and a fresh start. But we can build on it. As we focus on Him and claim His love and compassion and let Him fill us, then we have what we need to face each and every day.

In our health and fitness journey, we may exercise every day for several days and then we don't. Rest days are certainly good, but sometimes we miss a day just because we let life take over. We hit the snooze instead of getting up. But we have a chance the next day.

Maybe we make poor choices when it comes to our nutrition. Instead of letting a bad Monday turn into a bad week, we must get up on Tuesday and claim His strength and a fresh start on our nutrition.

If we take this promise carelessly, we just say "Oh well, I can keep starting over every day." But when is progress made? It's not. We can't make progress thinking that way.

He commits to us every day to bless us with a new day. We must be good stewards of that opportunity.

Prayer: Lord, today is a new day. Please be my portion and fill me with all I need to go through this day to glorify You. Thank You for Your love and compassion. I receive it now. Amen.

Action Step: Today's step takes a mindset shift. Let go of yesterday and face this day as the new day and new opportunity that this verse tells us it is. How will you seize it?

Journal

DAY 18

Psalm 139:13-17

Keep your eyes on your own paper.

No, this doesn't have anything to do with being in a classroom and taking a test. I'm referring to health and fitness plans and body image.

We have such a tendency to compare ourselves with others.

"She lost weight. I wonder how she did it?"

"Look at her. I wish I looked like that."

The Bible tells us we are "fearfully and wonderfully made." No two fingerprints are alike. We each have a unique DNA. So why would my plan for a healthy body look like your plan? And why would my uniquely and carefully crafted body look like yours?

Why would I want it to?

Let's take a look at a key passage in scripture:

> For You formed my inward parts; You covered me in
> my mother's womb.
> I will praise You , for I am *fearfully and wonderfully made*;
> marvelous are Your works, and that my soul knows
> very well.

My frame was not hidden from You, when I was *made in secret*,
and *skillfully* wrought in the lowest parts of the earth.
Your eyes saw my substance, being yet unformed.
And in Your book they all were written, the days fashioned *for me*.
When as yet there were none of them.
How *precious are Your thoughts about me*, O God!
How great is the sum of them!
Psalm 139: 13-17 (NKJV) (italics mine)

There are some key points in this verse that really jump out at me.

1. *fearfully and wonderfully made* - Do you see those words? You, I, we were fearfully and wonderfully made! This is with awe and excellence.
2. *made in secret* - I like to think that I was His own special secret. Before ANYONE knew that life had been created, before a test could show a positive result, HE knew I was there, because He already started forming me.
3. *skillfully* - This again refers to excellence, to something done well.
4. *precious are your thoughts about me* - And then He steps back and has only good thoughts of me. Precious refers to something highly valued. You and I are highly valued by our Creator.

Who are we to look in the mirror and judge what we see?

Yes, we should be good stewards of what we've been given.

Yes, we need to "eat to live, not live to eat" as Lysa TerKeurst writes.

But, health and fitness looks differently on and for everyone. This is why I plead with you "Keep your eyes on your own paper!" Stop looking! Stop trying to do something that will never work for you because you're not her...you're wonderful you!

Take the time to be a detective of your own body.

Doesn't it feel so much better when you turn in that assignment and know you can be confident in what's on your own paper?

You don't need to look at someone else's paper because you already know you got it right!

Prayer: Lord, help me see myself as the fearfully and wonderfully made creation that I am. Help me to honor the body You've given me. Thank You for knowing me before anyone else. I love You Lord. Amen.

Action Step: Look at the tips of your fingers. You have a unique fingerprint. Meditate on the thought that there is no one else exactly like you.

Journal

DAY 19

*"I have taught you in the way of wisdom; I have led you in the right paths. When you walk, your steps will not be hindered, and when you **run**, you will not stumble. Take firm hold of instruction, do not let go; keep her, for she is your life."* Proverbs 4:11-13 (NKJV)

I'm a runner. It's one of the first ways I and those who know me identify me. When I see the word "run," I perk up a little. In fact, it was a word of the year for me, not as in the physical aspect to run but in the spiritual aspect…to run the race marked out for me (Hebrews 12:1) and in such a way as to get the prize (I Corinthians 9:24).

So, when I read Proverbs 4 and saw the word "run," I took note.

Wisdom is available to us. We must ask for it. We can find it in God's Word. We have the Holy Spirit in us. We have fellow believers. He leads us on the right paths, and we have what we need.

So whether we are walking patiently on a journey He has placed us or we're running full speed ahead in a direction He is telling us to go, we can be sure that He will lead us there safely.

Yet don't miss that final verse: "take firm hold of instruction." This wisdom, this guidance, is our lifeline. I heard a pastor say that wisdom is our protection and that it brings a better type of life. But we must hold onto it. We need to grab it and not let it go.

Let's go back to running for a minute.

As a runner, one of the most important things for me is a good pair of running shoes. They can make or break how well I "survive" my workout. They protect my feet. Good shoes give me a better running experience.

So it is with wisdom, our protection, our lifeline. Wisdom helps us navigate the rocky paths. Wisdom helps us endure the obstacles life puts before us. Wisdom carries us to the mountaintops and supports us in the valley. If my shoes are on securely, I can walk through muddy trails without them coming off.

And so it is with wisdom…if I'm holding firmly, I can get through those rough patches by staying connected to the Lord. Wisdom keeps me on the right path.

The next time I lace up for my morning run, I'm going to consider how I'm choosing wisdom in my life and where I need to take firm hold of it.

How about you? Will you join me today and choose to take hold of wisdom and run where He's leading?

Prayer: Lord, I'm taking hold of Your hand. Guide me in wisdom. I will follow wherever You lead. In Jesus' name, Amen.

Action Step: Take a walk or go for a run. Tell the Lord you're ready to follow where He's leading.

Journal

DAY 20

"Present your bodies a living sacrifice, holy, acceptable to God, which is your reasonable service. And do not be conformed to this world, but be transformed by the renewing of your mind, that you may prove what is that good and acceptable and perfect will of God." Romans 12:1-2 (NKJV)

The first verse refers to the body and the second to the mind, yet they are connected. Your mind and your body. You can't let the world determine how either one works.

Our bodies are vessels for God to use and accomplish His work. They need to be healthy and strong so that we can complete the mission we've been given.

Our minds need to be set on things above and not on things here that distract. We cannot be comparing ourselves to others. We can't be seeking diets and quick fixes to get a body that looks like someone on a magazine cover.

God wants all of you. He wants you to believe the words He's written about your body and who you are in Him.

He wants us to care for our bodies and treat them with respect by exercising and feeding them healthy foods as well as appreciating how we are uniquely made.

One way that I can present my body to Him in worship is to make my daily workout an act of worship. I've always referred to my early morning run as my holy ground. It's when I meet with Him. I pray. I clear my mind. I listen for His voice. So many thoughts, answers, inspirations have come to me while I'm out on a run or a bike ride, just me and Him. Many of these entries and much of what I've ever shared in an email or blog post begins during a workout. It's a time when I feel close to Him.

How can you present yourself to Him as an act of worship? When do you feel closest to Him? Where is your holy ground?

Prayer: Lord, help me see that my body and mind belong to You. I come before You and present myself to You. Even though I may see myself as imperfect, You see me as perfect. You desire communion with me. Here I am Lord. Please use me. Amen.

Action Step: Approach your workout today as an act of worship. Play Christian music. Pray. Listen. Commit that time to Him.

Journal

DAY 21

"Do you not know that those who run in a race all run, but one receives the prize? Run in such a way that you may obtain it." 1 Corinthians 9:24 (NKJV)

I haven't won many races in my life. I've toed the line at more races than I can even keep track of. I've won my age group in a few, and I have been first female finisher in a few very small races. But I'm not an elite athlete by any stretch. Forever I've just called myself "an avid yet average runner."

But ask any runner. When a runner enters a race, he or she wants to do well. I know that I want to do well. The prize I'm shooting for may not be the overall prize, but it's to meet a goal I've set or maybe beat a time I've posted before.

In life, we are called to run a race. It's this race of life we've been placed in and set to run. And we are called to put forth our best effort at what He's called us to do.

That means wherever you are today and whatever you are doing. In your home. In your workplace. In your approach to your health and fitness.

You are where you are for a reason. Make today your best day.

Prayer: Lord, help me to keep my eye on the prize which is to bring You glory in what You've called me to do.

Show me how to train for the race before me. Thank You for cheering me on! Amen.

Action Step: Go for a run or a walk and think about the fact that you are running a race…your life, your calling. How are you doing? Do you need to set some goals? Do you need to push a little harder? How's your training plan?

Journal

DAY 22

"But I discipline my body and bring it into subjection…" 1 Corinthians 9:27 (NKJV)

Discipline in this case is not to be looked at as a negative thing. We see self-discipline as one of the fruits of the Spirit in Galatians. The Lord needs to be in control of all aspects of our lives down to how we spend our time and the things that we eat.

I'm not an advocate of counting calories or getting caught up with strict rules when it comes to eating and exercise; however, that does not give me clearance to eat however I want. If it were up to me, I would eat M&Ms all day long. While a few, perhaps even daily, would be considered fine, indulging in handfuls every day is not.

We need boundaries. We must discipline ourselves so as not to live carefree and end up being unhealthy and lethargic.

This could also pertain to your schedule. Are you staying up late watching television shows when you could be sleeping so that you're well-rested and your body has time to recover from the day? Are you hitting snooze instead of getting up for daily devotionals?

Exercise is important not only for weight loss but more importantly for a healthy heart, flexibility, energy, and longevity. It may not be something you *feel* like doing every day, but that's where discipline comes in. Getting up early if necessary even if we would prefer to lay in bed.

These are all examples of ways we need to discipline our bodies.

Prayer: Lord, help me to use the fruit of self-discipline in my life. This isn't about restricting and starving myself, but it is about not giving into the things that are not beneficial for my body. Help me to know the difference, Lord and to be faithful to honor the way You have created me. In Jesus' name, Amen.

Action Step: Talk to a trusted friend or coach who can help you look at your schedule and your nutrition to see if there is an area you can improve.

Journal

DAY 23

"I speak in human terms because of the weakness of your flesh. For just as you presented your members as slaves to uncleanness, and of lawlessness leading to more lawlessness, so now present your members as slaves of righteousness for holiness." Romans 6:19 (NKJV)

One translation says it more like this "...you are weak in your natural selves...you used to offer parts of your body in slavery to impurity…now offer them in slavery to righteousness…"

In her book <u>Made to Crave</u>, Lysa TerKeurst writes "these boundaries are in place for our freedom."

We often tell small children they can play in our fenced-in yard. They have the freedom to roam anywhere *within* the safety of the fence. Those boundaries are there for their safety. They can run free and still stay safe. If we let our child run out the front door, he may be free but he is not safe. Then fear and danger set in.

It's the same with our health and fitness. We may have access to all types of food, but it's not in our best interest to eat it all. It's not healthy for our bodies. Maybe we need to journal what we eat or track it with something like Calorie King to help us learn how many and what kinds of calories our bodies need.*

When we're training for an event, we need to follow a training plan. If we want to run a half marathon, we need to be prepared to cover the distance. We have the freedom to choose our pace, but if we have chosen that distance we need to add the mileage regularly and safely.

Our victory depends on staying within the safe boundaries He has set for us.

Prayer: Lord, thank You for keeping me safe in Your arms. Thank You for loving me enough to give me boundaries. Help me to honor them so that I'm always safe in Your care. In Your name I pray, Amen.

Action Step: Do you need to set some boundaries? Assess your health and fitness.

*Please be sure, I only suggest this for educational purposes. I'm the first to tell you that I have gotten caught up in all these numbers and they became a distraction. This is not a long-term solution by any means. I only suggest this if you are new to understanding the nutritional value of food.

Journal

DAY 24

"Then you will walk safely in your way, and your foot will not stumble." Proverbs 3:23 (NKJV)

Prior to this verse, we read about wisdom and understanding. We must be seeking those things *so that* we "walk safely…and not stumble."

We can use this verse in life as it relates to following the path we're on. I have also used this as scripture for healing. As a runner, I have been injured. Most of the time it's something nagging that doesn't completely sideline me but makes running uncomfortable. If the injury is stressed, it can lead to long layoffs.

A few years ago I was getting ready to run a half marathon, and I had a foot injury. (I referenced this back in Day 9.) I was searching scripture for a verse I could claim through the run. One that would speak directly to that foot. And so I prayed and the Lord led me to this verse. I wrote it on a notecard. I took it with me in the car on race morning. I memorized it. I ran that race without pain and without further injury. I did have to baby the foot for a few days after the race, but He gave me what I needed when I needed it.

He is faithful. Even those things that you think are minor or that you think you shouldn't be asking for because they seem selfish are important. If something is important to you, it's important to Him. He wants us to go to Him for everything! Every single thing! What do you need to take to Him today? Nothing is too small.

Prayer: Lord, here I am. Thank You for taking the time to listen to my prayers and requests. I know that I'm important to You and that what is going on with me is important to You. Here are my concerns today. Please help me. Amen.

Action Step: Take your concerns to Him. Write down your requests and keep track of how He shows up.

Journal

DAY 25

"For you are the temple of the living God." 2 Corinthians 6:16 (NKJV)

I know we've covered this before. We've talked about the fact that you are a temple - not a trash can.

Sometimes we need to hear this more than once. If it's in the Bible more than once in more than one way, then it must be something we need to get.

So, how are you doing? It's been a couple of weeks since we first addressed this issue. Has it made a difference in the way that you are treating your body? In the way that you look at yourself?

In fact, let's talk more about that. The first time we talked about how we treated our bodies. Temple vs. Trash Can.

But today, let's talk about how you *view* it. That's a bit different.

I don't know about you; but when I see a beautiful building, I'm in awe. I think about all it took to make it look as such. I think about the intricate details. Think of a church or cathedral or museum you've gone into. Maybe there were stained glass windows or ornate woodwork.

Did you just stand back and take it all in with amazement of all it took to create such a thing?

Did you know that you and I are just as amazing? We were created with great care and attention to detail.

So I ask you again, how are you doing treating your body like a temple? Can you stand and look at your reflection in the mirror and be in awe of what you see?

Prayer: Dear Lord, thank You for creating me with such care and detail. Thank You for how amazing my body is. Please help me to look at my reflection with the same awe that You do. Amen.

Action Step: Go stand in front of the mirror and identify something unique and beautiful about you. It might be a birthmark or your eyes or a dimple in your cheek. It's there. Don't leave until you notice it.

Journal

DAY 26

"But indeed, O man, who are you to reply against God? Will the thing formed say to him who formed it, 'Why have you made me like this?'" Romans 9:20 (NKJV)

How many times have I looked in the mirror and pointed out what was wrong with me? Anyone else?

My breasts aren't the right size.

I wish I had a flat stomach.

If I could only grow an inch or two.

How am I ever going to get some shape to my flat behind?

Have you ever had any of these thoughts or conversations *with yourself* in the mirror?

But wait. Conversations *with yourself…* Well, you may be alone, but are you? You may think you're just talking to your reflection, but are you?

Sweet sister, you are a created being. Someone formed you. Someone created you to be just as you are.

I would suggest that this conversation you're having is more than just with the person staring back at you. It is with the Creator Himself. He hears you and knows what you're saying.

Ok, maybe you haven't been the best steward of the body you've been given. Maybe there are some healthy choices you need to start making. But the bottom line is this: He made you exactly the way you were supposed to be made.

When your child brings you his artwork, do you look at him and tell him you don't like it? Do you tell him it wasn't supposed to be made that way? That his way isn't how it's supposed to be?

Of course you don't! You cherish his artwork. In fact, you find a special place to display it for ALL to see.

In the same way, our Creator has said "here is this body for you, wonderfully made, just for you to care for."

Prayer: Thank You, Lord, for making me just the way I'm supposed to be. Thank You for crafting me into a beautiful woman. Help me be a good steward with that which You have entrusted me. Amen.

Action Step: Take a selfie and hang it on your refrigerator or display it somewhere that you and others can see. Be grateful for how you have been fashioned today.

Journal

DAY 27

"And He said to me, 'My grace is sufficient for you, for My strength is made perfect in weakness.' Therefore most gladly I will rather boast in my infirmities, that the power of Christ may rest upon me. Therefore I take pleasure in infirmities, in reproaches, in needs, in persecutions, in distresses, for Christ's sake. For when I am weak, then I am strong." 2 Corinthians 12:9-10 (NKJV)

I've always said that my struggles with weight, self-image, negative self-talk, etc., are what has kept me on my knees. And as much as I coach and counsel women, I have times when I still struggle. I find myself wanting to find a quick fix or taking 20 pictures before posting one I feel good about or NOT posting a picture at all because I just don't feel good about how I look. Yet, I keep tackling this head on every day, and some days I'm living totally "fit and free," but other days it takes everything in me to believe my own stuff.

The struggle may never go away completely, and sometimes I have to think that it's not supposed to…

You see, we need Him. But sometimes it's easy to ignore Him or forget when things seem to be going okay.

I'm blessed. I have periods of my life that seem to be going just fine, but no matter what is happening, this struggle with my weight and body image is always very close to the surface. It's reared its ugly head so many times that I know I have to start each day asking for help in this area and surrendering it, and I still don't get it right each time. But it keeps me at His feet.

Yours may be the same, or it may be something different. I'm not sure what your ongoing struggle is. Instead of wishing it away, thank Him for it. Let it be that thing that keeps you closely connected to Him.

Prayer: Lord, I know You are strong in me. I rely on Your strength every single day. Thank You for drawing me to You and giving me a new dose of Your strength. I don't want to ever drift far away from Your presence. In Your precious name, Amen.

Action Step: Go to the mirror and make a muscle. Thank God for the strength He gives you today and every day.

Journal

DAY 28

"Let not your heart be troubled; you believe in God, believe also in Me." John 14:1 (NKJV)

How often do we get all worked up about our struggles with weight loss and fitness?

I have cried WAY too many tears over a number on a scale. I've scoured the internet for weight loss plans and pills that would help me lose those last five pounds. I have allowed myself to get so troubled over my body size.

In fact, I remember a specific time I had a horrible day because I wore something that was a little snug and all day long I was thinking it was a bigger size than it was. When I took it off and realized it was the smaller size, I didn't feel so bad.

How many times have we created trouble or stress that isn't even true???

This passage tells us "let NOT your heart be troubled." If I believe in God then I should know that He has a plan for me. He has created me the way that I am. I may need to change a few habits to become a bit healthier, but I can't let myself get overwhelmed with things like a few pounds.

I believe He created me. I believe that He loves me. I believe that I am fearfully and wonderfully made.

How about you? What do you believe? Is your heart

troubled in this area of health and fitness? It's time to give it over to Him. Believe in Him. He's got this.

Prayer: Lord, calm my spirit, quiet my mind. Help me to be open to the truth of Your Word which tells me that I am fearfully and wonderfully made and that I only need to believe in and rely on You. In Jesus' name, Amen.

Action Step: If the numbers on the scale are causing your spirit to be troubled, get rid of them. Whatever it is that you are obsessing about and that is causing worry, get that out of your life. If it's a magazine cover, toss the magazine. Go to Him instead.

Journal

DAY 29

"For we are His workmanship, created in Christ Jesus for good works, which God prepared beforehand that we should walk in them." Ephesians 2:10 (NKJV)

I looked up *workmanship* on dictionary.com. It says "it is the product or result of labor and skill." I don't know about you, but that makes me feel pretty special.

You and I took labor and skill to become who we are. The Creator took care and concern to make you and me.

Synonyms for workmanship include "artwork" and "expertise." Wow! You are a picture of His expertise. You are a piece of artwork. AND, He has prepared something for you to do. There is a plan for me and for you that will utilize the unique qualities He's given each of us.

Have you thought of yourself in these terms? How special and unique you are? And that there is something special and specific for you to do? Do you know what it is? Are you seeking Him to find out what it is He wants you to do?

Prayer: Lord, show me what You have prepared for me to do. Thank You for taking care to make me unique so that I might be prepared to do the things which You have called me to do. In Your name I pray, Amen.

Action Step: Look at your life, your talents and abilities.

Are you using them for Him? What steps do you need to take to walk on the path and in the plan He has for you?

Journal

DAY 30

"And Jabez called on the God of Israel saying, 'Oh, that You would bless me indeed, and enlarge my territory, that Your hand would be with me, and that You would keep me from evil, that I may not cause pain!' So God granted him what he requested." 1 Chronicles 4:10 (NKJV)

The Prayer of Jabez. It has been taught and preached about. I believe there has even been a book written with the same title expanding upon it. It's something I have on a notecard and pray regularly. I want to share some of those notes I have. I've had it so long that I'm not sure whom to give credit to, but I know I heard a message on this topic.

Bless me - We ask for God's blessing on our lives so we can glorify Him. All good things come from Him. Any blessing we receive should be used for His glory.

Enlarge my territory - We want to reach as many as we can in His name. Asking for our territory to enlarge is asking to grow our ministry and our reach. No matter where you are planted, you have a ministry.

That Your hand would be upon me - This is a request for His power, wisdom, and anointing to do what it is He has called us to do. We don't want to move or do anything outside of His will or on our own power.

Keep me from evil - Pray to be surrounded by His protection. He is our Good Shepherd. He watches over us.

What business are you about? What is your work or your vocation? What is your calling? You may work in a factory or drive a semi. You may sit at a desk and answer phones or oversee a large corporation. You might be a stay-at-home mom or a work-at-home mom. Maybe you're a student or retired.

Whatever it is that you do, dedicate it to Him. Pray over it and ask that He maximize your work and that He be glorified in the process.

Prayer: Lord, thank You for the way that You have already blessed my life. I ask that I use all blessings for Your glory. Increase my reach and my ministry. May all that I do have Kingdom impact. Give me strength and guidance, and empower me with Your Spirit to do all that You are calling me to. And please surround me with Your hedge of protection. Thank You in advance for what You're doing in me and through me. Amen.

Action Step: Write this prayer on a notecard and begin to pray and believe that He is going to do mighty things through you.

Journal

DAY 31

"For the Lord your God is a consuming fire, a jealous God." Deuteronomy 4:24 (NKJV)

God loves you. He wants all of you.

As a woman, doesn't it feel just a little bit good when your husband or boyfriend gets kind of jealous? (I'm not talking anything major or extreme!) Maybe you dress up to go out, and he says something like "Stay close to me tonight. I want everyone to know you're with me." Or you're meeting a girlfriend for dinner, and he notices how nice you look and says something like "I wish I were going out with you."

The point here is this: God is a jealous God. He wants all of us. He wants our full hearts. He wants our passion and desire to be for Him. To follow Him. To obey Him. To represent Him to a lost and dying world.

When we are distracted by other things…whether they be feelings of insecurity and inadequacy or sinful behaviors…He is sad. He does not like to see His children wandering and giving their attention to things that He has not meant for us to.

Too much of my time and attention was being wasted worrying about a number on a scale or how many calories I had left to eat on a certain day or if I should do a second workout to burn x number of calories.

On those days, and during those seasons of my life, He was jealous. He wanted my focus to be on Him, not on a number on a scale. He wanted me to be about the business of sharing His love with others and accepting the love He had for me.

His desire is that we are consumed with His love for us.

What is consuming you today? Let His love consume you.

Prayer: Lord, I love You. Thank You for loving me so much that You want all of me. Help me set the distractions aside and focus on You. It's in Your name I pray, Amen.

Action Step: God's Word is His love letter to you. Spend some time reading the Bible today and let His love consume you. John 3:16 may be a good place to start with.

Journal

DAY 32

"Do not let any unwholesome talk come out of your mouths but only what is helpful for building others up according to their needs, that it may benefit those who listen." Ephesians 4:29 (NIV)

Oh the words that we speak…

You know the saying "Sticks and stones may break my bones but words will never hurt me"?

Just raise your hand if you completely disagree with that statement! (I'm raising my hand for sure!)

When I was in high school, I was sitting on my front porch with a boy who (supposedly) liked me when he told me 'You know, somebody once told me never to judge a book by its cover." And I'm sitting there trying to figure out what he was saying. Well, he didn't leave me hanging very long. He then said "You know, you're not that pretty…" I can't recall what he said after that. Maybe something about how nice I am or that I was quiet and hard to get to know. To this day, I can't remember the rest of the conversation. But I can tell you this: I would've rather had someone throw sticks at me at that moment than tell me something like that. Especially given that he thought he was giving me a compliment!!

Words.

One year my word for the year was "Beneficial." One of the areas I applied it to was my words. I always spent much time worrying about what I put *into* my mouth, but that year I wanted to apply it also to what came *out* of my mouth. I began to take a minute before I responded to something. I tried to slow myself down before I spoke to my husband and my sons, especially when it involved a chore forgotten or a mess left behind.

Our words have an impact.

What about the words you say to the person looking back at you in the mirror? Do you pick out every flaw? Do you tell that person she isn't good enough, pretty enough, committed enough? Are you always telling her what's wrong with her and what she didn't do right?

Our words are meant to be encouraging and uplifting. They need to be beneficial to those who hear them whether that be your friends and family, a stranger behind the grocery counter, or the reflection in the mirror.

How are your words?

Prayer: Dear Lord, may my words benefit all who listen. Help me to be slow to speak. When I do, let me speak words of life and goodness. Amen.

Action Step: Pick your words carefully today. Tell your family that you love them and tell them something you appreciate about them. Go to the mirror and say something kind to the person looking back at you.

Journal

DAY 33

"No temptation has overtaken you except such as is common to man; but God is faithful, who will not allow you to be tempted beyond what you are able, but with the temptation will also make the way of escape, that you may be able to bear it." 1 Corinthians 10:13 (NKJV)

We are going to be tempted. Everywhere we turn, we face temptation. Healthy living can be tough. There are ads for 2-for-1 Quarter Pounders, and every drive thru gives you the option to supersize!

If you live with anyone, whether it's one person or a full household, you know that everyone has various tastes and health needs and not all people under the same roof may subscribe to the way you are choosing to eat or to the lifestyle changes you want to make. And that's okay.

What we know is that there will be temptations, but God is faithful to give us the strength to say no to those things that are not beneficial to us. When we remember why we are doing what we're doing and how good we feel when we pass up the chips or the extra helpings, then we will be able to make the right choice.

Is it easy? Not always, but with Christ we have the strength. Remember, He was tempted and overcame.

Prayer: Lord give me the strength to say no when temptation comes my way. I know it won't always be easy, but You always reward obedience. I want to choose You and Your ways. Thank You for the strength You give and the example You set. Amen.

Action Step: The next time you feel you need to say No to something, switch your perspective and put a positive spin on it. For example, instead of "I can't have those Reese's Cups," say "I'm making my chocolate protein shake with some peanut butter and that is going to give me the satisfaction AND the energy I need today." If you're tempted to hit the snooze button, instead recognize it as an opportunity for some time to yourself before everyone else gets up.

Journal

DAY 34

"We are carefully joined together in Him, becoming a holy temple for the Lord." Ephesians 2:21 (NLT)

There are several references in scripture about how we are a temple…our bodies are a temple or the temple of the Lord. We see temple referenced here yet again. But for this verse, I want to focus on the first part *"we are carefully joined together."*

I love women! I love the community of women. I love going on bike rides with my "girlfriends" and studying the Bible in a women's Bible study. I love to call myself a woman. And yet competition and comparison can rear its ugly head among women. I know firsthand!

I remember constantly comparing myself to other girls when I was growing up, sometimes even to my closest friends. While they were my friends, this comparison would give me this sense of competition. I wanted to be prettier and more liked than she. I wanted a boy to pick me over her.

And even as women, let's be honest, we'll size ourselves up with other women. How many times have you been out, possibly already feeling self-conscious for one reason or another, and then someone walks into the restaurant and you begin the comparisons in your mind?

I'm raising my hand. I've done it. It could be a stranger or it could be a close friend.

But here's the thing: we're in this together! We're all part of this life together. If the Lord lives in your heart as He does mine, we're sisters in Christ. We can't let this comparison and competition take over. We're supposed to be lifting one another up and encouraging each other.

I used to think that if I complimented someone, then I was in turn putting myself down. Or if my friend had success in some area, be it job or weight loss or whatever, it meant failure for me.

That is so not right! How is it that we come to think this way?

As the verse says "we," *we* - you and me sister - we're joined together. We're in this together. And we're *all* a temple of the Lord.

Prayer: Dear God, please remove any spirit of comparison or competition from my heart. I want to be supportive of the beautiful women around me. Thank You for making me a woman. Help me to encourage the community of women and help us to be confident in the unique way that you have made each of us. In Jesus' name I pray, Amen.

Action Step: Give a genuine compliment to a female friend or stranger today.

Journal

DAY 35

"Stand fast therefore in the liberty by which Christ has made us free, and do not be entangled again with a yoke of bondage." Galatians 5:1 (NKJV)

Stand in liberty. Christ paid the price for us to be free. Free from sin. Free from bondage.

Sister, there was a time in my life when all I wanted was freedom. I knew that I was bound with negative self-talk. I was bound up in comparison and competition with everyone I looked at. I felt inferior and not good enough. I just wanted to be free.

As I did Beth Moore's study "Breaking Free," I began to learn what it meant to walk in freedom in Christ. I began to appreciate the price that He paid. I learned that it was ME who allowed myself to remain in bondage. I was a Christ follower, but I was not accepting the freedom that was already mine in Christ.

Is there an area of your life that you feel tied up? An area that you feel as if you will never shake but you so want to be free? He paid the price.

How many of us walk by a freebie in a store? I doubt many of us. Even if we don't *need* it, we take it because, well, it's free of course!

This is free AND you need it. I need it. Christ paid for my freedom and yours. He's standing there offering it to you today.

Prayer: Lord, I want to be free. I want to walk in the freedom that You bought for me. This bondage is unnecessary. It's self-inflicted. I receive the freedom that is mine. I'm going to walk in freedom today. Thank You for setting me free. Amen.

Action Step: Lift your hands in praise to the Lord. Sing a song of thanksgiving. Run or dance around your house. Practice freedom!

Journal

DAY 36

"The secret things belong to the Lord our God, but those things that are revealed belong to us and to our children forever, that we may do all the words of this law." Deuteronomy 29:29 (NKJV)

This is Old Testament scripture and written before Christ was revealed. There was so much yet to come. However, the people of God had been given His law and promises of things yet to come.

We don't know everything yet to come in our lives, but we know the One who does. We have His Word…His full and complete Word. We have our life experiences of how He has shown up in our lives and blessed us and answered our prayers and been with us through good and bad times. We know how He has been faithful to save us from our sin and to lead us into a life that is everlasting.

I'm not sure what you are facing right now. You may have a big decision to make. You may be sick or in pain and not know how, when, or if the healing will come.

We don't always know everything, but we know God's Word. It is truth. It is what we can rely on. It's the truth we need to share in our homes and with our children.

He just asks that we obey His commands and trust His Word.

Prayer: Dear Lord, I trust You. I may not know everything I'd like to right now, but I know You are faithful. I know Your Word is true. Give me peace for this day. Thank You for Your faithfulness to me yesterday, today, and always. In Your name I pray, Amen.

Action Step: Take some quiet time in His Word. Find a promise and write it down on a notecard and remind yourself that He is in control. He knows the end of the story.

Journal

DAY 37

"Rejoice always, pray without ceasing, in everything give thanks; for this is the will of God in Christ Jesus for you." I Thessalonians 5:16-18 (NKJV)

Rejoice always. According to Dictionary.com, rejoice means to delight in or be glad. It's about attitude.

Pray without ceasing. When Ethan was small, he would stop everything and pray. I once saw him on the soccer field as a little guy close his eyes and pray. As precious as that is, that is not what this means. (God doesn't want us to get hit in the head with a soccer ball!)

We can be in a spirit of prayer all the time, having our minds and thoughts focused on Christ, including Him in all that we do. It may be a "thank You, Jesus" when something good happens. Or a "Lord, please help me" during a tough time or a split-second decision you need to make. It's about where our heart is focused.

In everything, give thanks. We must have a grateful heart. Having a gratitude journal is a great way to keep your focus towards gratitude. It only takes a couple minutes at the end of each day to write down something for which you are grateful. It could be as simple as a mug of hot chocolate on a winter evening or as significant as a job promotion.

For this is the will of God…for you. This is how He wants us to live. He wants us to maintain a positive outlook because we're seeking Him and trusting Him *for* all things and *in* all things.

Prayer: Lord, I come to You today to focus my mind and my heart on You. Help me not to take that focus away. Give me a heart of gratitude that trusts that Your ways are good. Amen.

Action Step: Begin a gratitude journal. Write down three things at the end of the day for which you are thankful.

Journal

DAY 38

"But the Lord said to Samuel, "Do not look at his appearance or at his physical stature, because I have refused him. For the Lord does not see as man sees, for man looks at the outward appearance, but the Lord looks at the heart." 1 Samuel 16:7 (NKJV)

Aren't you glad that the Lord does not judge us on looks? Or are you? Maybe you put a lot of work into what your outer self looks like, but maybe it's what's on the inside that needs a little sprucing up?

Our society is so focused on what we see. There is so much attention paid to outward appearance. But this isn't new. We're reading this in the Old Testament. It was time to choose the next king, so Samuel would've likely looked for a strong man, someone who walked with confidence and authority. But the Lord said "No." That wasn't what He was looking at. He was looking at the condition of the man's heart.

Our first response to this verse is often the feeling that we're off the hook. We might be thinking "I'm nothing to look at on the outside. Thank goodness God said not to judge on outward appearance." But there is that heart condition. And sometimes my heart condition doesn't look so great. I might be harboring ill feelings or thoughts towards someone. I may have engaged in gossip or judgement.

How's the condition of your heart? Are you taking as much time working on that as you do on hair and makeup and your daily workout? I had to start setting my alarm a bit earlier so I wouldn't rush through my Bible study just to get out on my run or to get on with my day.

He's interested in your heart.

Prayer: Lord, it's so easy to read this verse and say "Well, I'm not pretty by society's standards so thank You for not focusing on the outward," but then we miss the part about the heart. My heart isn't always pure and right, and I need You. I need You to check my heart and heal my heart. I ask this in Your name, Amen.

Action Step: Write this verse on a notecard and post it to your bathroom mirror. Use it as a reminder of what is important to the Lord. Set an intention to set your heart towards Him on a daily basis.

Journal

DAY 39

"Be strong and of good courage, do not fear or be afraid of them; for the Lord your God, He is the One who goes with you. He will not leave you nor forsake you." Deuteronomy 31:6 (NKJV)

Worry. How many times have you let it take over your thoughts and emotions? Too many times to count? Me too.

Dictionary.com defines the act of worrying this way: to torment oneself with or suffer from disturbing thoughts; fret. *Torment.* That's a strong word. *Suffer disturbing thoughts.* This doesn't sound good. In fact, there's not much good that can come from worrying except to get our focus off of God and onto ourselves and our circumstances and then allow it to disrupt the rest of our lives.

I spent hours, days, years worrying about my appearance. Worrying about the number on the scales. Worrying about what I would order when we went to a restaurant. Worrying if someone would look at me and think I had gained weight. Worry, worry, worry.

Did the worry make me more attractive? Did it help me lose weight? Did it change what I ate at the restaurant? Did it affect how people saw me?

The only thing worry did was exhaust me. It kept my focus on ME instead of my calling and my purpose and the people in my life.

As God's people, we are called to be strong and courageous. We can be brave and confident because our God is with us. He's got us.

Are you allowing yourself to be consumed with worry? Whether it's about your pant size or your children or a job?

Worry can attack us from any angle and many angles all at once. But we don't have to let it consume us. When it comes, we have to take it to the Lord. We have to claim the promise in this verse that He is with us. There is nothing that we need to fear.

Prayer: Lord, I'm laying down this worry at Your feet. It's distracted me far too long. In its place I'm claiming victory. I am no longer afraid of this situation. You are on my side, and I know that's all I need. Please take this Lord and give me strength to move beyond this worry and instead walk in courage. I'm trusting You today, Amen.

Action Step: Lift some weights today. If you don't have weights, find something heavy to lift. Grab the milk jug, some cans of soup, a brick that's in the garage (don't hurt yourself though!). As you're lifting them, think of how strong you are and how much strength you have in Christ.

Journal

DAY 40

"Therefore whether you eat or drink or whatever you do, do all to the glory of God." I Corinthians 10:31 (NKJV)

This has been a life verse for me. It sums up everything I'm about. It takes into consideration the minor details and the big picture.

Whatever you do…do it for God's glory.

As you consider your life and how you're living for God, know that even what you eat and drink matters to Him. How you treat your body matters to Him. Our eating and drinking can glorify Him or not.

When we refuse to care for our bodies, we're refusing to care for His creation.

When we don't consider what we're putting in our bodies, we're forgetting that we are fearfully and wonderfully made.

When you buy a car, you put the right kind of fuel in it, don't you? You wouldn't put vegetable oil in your car and expect it to perform at its best right? If you did and you're stuck on the side of the road, what are people going to think when you tell them you put vegetable oil in the fuel tank? They might question your intelligence!

The same goes with us. How we treat our bodies matters to God and it says something about what we believe about

Him. He put care and concern in creating us. He loves us. We want to be living examples of that and be able to share Him with others.

Are you eating and drinking in a way that glorifies God?

Prayer: Lord, whatever I do, whether I eat or drink, I want to glorify You. Please show me how to do that. Please show me ways to care for myself that brings You glory and honor. Help my life be a blessing to You Lord. Amen.

Action Step: Put this verse on the refrigerator. Let it be a reminder that everything we do should bring glory to God.

Journal

EPILOGUE

Your 40 days may be ending, but your faith and fitness journey continues. My prayer for every woman who reads this book and gets to this page is that she, that you Sister, will know that you have been fearfully and wonderfully made and loved just as you are.

I pray that you now see yourself as Christ sees you and as a result you will live to honor Him in all that you do including caring for your body which is a temple of His Holy Spirit.

I hope that throughout these pages you've heard the message that a fit life and a healthy life doesn't look the same for everyone. You have been carefully crafted and uniquely created. Therefore, your healthy lifestyle and fit body won't look like your sister's, but that's okay, and that's the beautiful thing about how we have been created.

May you continue on this path of faith and fitness by keeping your eyes on your Maker and living each day with the confidence that you are a daughter of a King.

ABOUT THE AUTHOR

Marsha Apsley desires to live according to 1 Corinthians 10:31 "So whether you eat or drink or whatever you do, do it all for the glory of God." She believes that God wants to be part of our everyday lives including how we eat and drink and how we view our reflection in the mirror. She's cried far too many tears over a number on a scale but is thankful that God can use those experiences to help other women.

Marsha is a counselor and is passionate about helping women live fit and free. She does this by focusing on whole person health and wellness with an emphasis on how women feel about themselves. She believes that a healthy lifestyle needs to be built on a firm foundation of faith.

She is a wife and mom of two sons. She loves to run and bike and enjoy a cup of coffee with friends. She believes every day is better when it includes a little chocolate.

For support and encouragement on your faith and fitness journey, please visit her website www.marshaapsley.com or find her on social media @marshaapsley. If you'd like to be part of a tribe of women who are building a healthy life on a foundation of faith, join Marsha's free Facebook group Faith and Fitness with Marsha. It's a sisterhood of women who have found we are stronger together. The doors are always open. To contact Marsha to speak at your next event, email her at marsha@marshaapsley.com.

Made in the USA
Monee, IL
07 July 2021